STAY SAFE FROM MONKEYPOX

what you should know about Monkeypox disease

Dr Aaron Hanson

CONTENT

What are the risk factors for monkeypox?

DESCRIPTION

The clinical appearance of monkeypox mirrors that of smallpox, a similar orthopoxvirus illness that has been eliminated. Smallpox was more readily spread and more frequently lethal as roughly 30 percent of patients perished. The final instance of spontaneously acquired smallpox occurred in 1977, and in 1980 smallpox was reported to have been eliminated globally following a global campaign of vaccination and containment. It has been 40 or more years since all nations halted regular smallpox immunization using vaccinia-based vaccines. As immunization also protected against monkeypox in west and central Africa, unvaccinated populations are now more vulnerable to monkeypox virus infection.

Whereas smallpox no longer occurs naturally, the global health sector remains attentive in the case it may resurface by natural causes, laboratory accidents, or purposeful release. To assure worldwide preparation in the case of a reemergence of smallpox, additional vaccinations, diagnostics, and antiviral medicines are being developed. These may also now be effective for the prevention and control of monkeypox.

This book born out of research contains all you need to know about Monkeypox disease; how it started, how to identify the disease, how it spreads, symptoms, prevention and many more.

INTRODUCTION

Monkeypox is a viral zoonosis (an infection sent to people from creatures) with side effects like those found in the past in smallpox patients, even though it is clinically less serious. With the destruction of smallpox in 1980 and the ensuing end of smallpox immunization, monkeypox has arisen as the most significant orthopoxvirus for general wellbeing. Monkeypox fundamentally happens in focal and west

Africa, frequently in nearness to tropical rainforests, and has been progressively showing up in metropolitan regions. The creature has incorporated a scope of rodents and non-human primates.

THE MICROORGANISM

Monkeypox infection is an encompassed twofold abandoned DNA infection that has a place with the Orthopoxvirus class of the Poxviridae family. There are two unmistakable hereditary clades of the monkeypox infection: the focal African (Congo Basin) clade and the west African clade. The Congo Basin clade has generally caused more extreme sickness and was believed to be more contagious. The geological division between the two clades has so far been in Cameroon, the main nation where both infection clades have been found.

Normal host of monkeypox infection

Different creature species have been distinguished as vulnerable to monkeypox infection. This incorporates rope squirrels, tree squirrels, Gambian pouched rodents, dormice, non-human primates, and different species. Vulnerability stays on the normal history of monkeypox infection and further examinations are expected to distinguish the specific reservoir(s) and how the infection course is kept up within nature.

Flare-ups

Human monkeypox was first recognized in quite a while in 1970 in the Democratic Republic of the Congo in a 9-month-old kid in a locale where smallpox had been disposed of in 1968. From that point forward, most cases have been accounted for from the country, rainforest districts of the Congo Basin, especially in the Democratic Republic of the Congo, and human cases have progressively been accounted for from across focal and west Africa.

Starting around 1970, human instances of monkeypox have

been accounted for in 11 African nations: Benin, Cameroon, the Central African Republic, the Democratic Republic of the Congo, Gabon, Côte d'Ivoire, Liberia, Nigeria, the Republic of the Congo, Sierra Leone, and South Sudan. The genuine weight of monkeypox isn't known. For instance, in 1996-97, a flare-up was accounted for in the Democratic Republic of the Congo with a lower case casualty proportion and a higher assault rate than expected.

A simultaneous flare-up of chickenpox (brought about by

the varicella infection, which isn't an orthopoxvirus) and monkeypox were found, which could make sense of genuine or obvious changes in transmission elements for this situation. Beginning around 2017, Nigeria has encountered an enormous episode, with north of 500 thought cases and more than 200 affirmed cases, and a case casualty proportion of roughly 3%. Cases keep on being accounted for until the present time.

Monkeypox is a sickness of worldwide general wellbeing significance as it not just influences nations in the west and focal Africa, yet the remainder of the world. In 2003, the first monkeypox episode beyond Africa was in the United States of America and was connected to contact with contaminated pet grassland canines.

These pets had been housed with Gambian pouched rodents and dormice that had been brought into the country from

Ghana. This episode prompted more than 70 instances of monkeypox in the U.S. Monkeypox has likewise been accounted for in voyagers from Nigeria to Israel in September 2018, to the United Kingdom in September 2018, December 2019, May 2021, and May 2022, to Singapore in May 2019, and to the United States of America in July and November 2021.

In May 2022, numerous instances of monkeypox were distinguished in a few non-endemic nations. Studies are in progress to additionally figure out the study of disease transmission, wellsprings of contamination, and transmission designs.

Further history of monkeypox including the 2022 flare-up

Monkeypox has a moderately ongoing history. Individuals originally found it in monkeys in 1958, albeit a "vesicular sickness in monkeys" was depicted during the 1860s. The illness, and ultimately the causative infection, was named monkeypox because the sores (pox) found in monkeys created like other known pox-framing sicknesses (pustules that at last tear open, ulcerate, hull over, and some pox structure scars in the skin).

Later examinations showed the "monkeypox" infection was supported endemically in African rodents. It was only after 1970 in Africa (Zaire, presently the Democratic Republic of Congo additionally named Republic of the Congo, DRC, and Congo) when a 9-year-old kid (who created smallpox-like sores) was the principal individual ultimately determined to have monkeypox. This present circumstance at first caused worry that smallpox may likewise have a creature repository or endemic populace that would make the destruction of smallpox incomprehensible.

Luckily, this was not the case because monkeypox was viewed as an alternate type of poxvirus, and smallpox was killed by the human populace by immunizations in 1979 (right now, a couple of examination labs approach smallpox infections). Monkeypox is presently the major

Orthopoxvirus (likewise named orthopox) that contaminates people and luckily, not habitually. Notwithstanding, watchfulness is justified, as there have been a few flare-ups of monkeypox since the 1970s. Albeit most have happened in Africa (chiefly western and focal Africa), there was a flare-up in the U.S. in 2003.

This happened when a creature merchant either housed or moved monkeypox-contaminated African rodents (Gambian rodents) with grassland canines that individuals later bought as pets, became "wiped out," and sent the sickness to their proprietors. Different creatures like the rope squirrel (Funisciurus anerythrus) and the sun squirrel (Heliosciurus rufobrachium) may communicate the infection to people in Africa.

In 2017, a flare-up of monkeypox started in Nigeria. This huge episode is believed to be set off by waterway flooding that has caused tainted wild creatures (particularly rodents and monkeys) to all the more intently partner with people, accordingly spreading this zoonotic (sent to people from creatures) sickness. From 2017 to the present, Nigeria has recorded 446 cases. In September 2018, Dr. Beadsworth in England detailed treating three individuals with monkeypox who had visited Nigeria. The three patients probably presented with the infection while visiting Nigeria. On July 15, 2021, an individual was determined to have monkeypox in Dallas, Texas, and the CDC affirmed this. He went via air from Nigeria to Atlanta,

Georgia, and afterward flew on to Dallas, Texas. The two carriers he utilized had required veils, so the CDC thinks the gamble is low for transmission of the sickness. One more case was analyzed in Maryland in 2021.

The ongoing flare-up (May 2022) has spread to non-endemic nations as to the World Health Organization (WHO). The nations incorporate Australia, Belgium, Canada, France, Germany, Italy, Netherlands, Portugal, Spain, Sweden, the United Kingdom

(Britain), and the USA. Most cases (around 21-30 for every nation) are in Spain, Portugal, and the United Kingdom. Furthermore, Israel, Switzerland, Denmark, and the Canary Islands have announced something like one affirmed case. Different nations presently can't seem to archive their cases. The U.S. has a few hypothetical cases recognized in voyagers to Florida with one affirmed; Massachusetts, New York, Utah, and Washington all have a most un-one recorded case.

HOW IT SPREADS

TRANSMISSION

Monkeypox spreads fundamentally through direct contact with irresistible injuries, scabs, or body liquids, including during sex, as well as exercises can imagine kissing, embracing, kneading, and nestling. Monkeypox can spread through contacting materials utilized by an individual with monkeypox that hasn't been cleaned, like clothing and bedding. It can likewise spread by respiratory emissions during drawn-out, close, eye-to-eye contact.

Precisely how is the infection spreading?

Toward the start of the flare-up, wellbeing authorities attested that the infection spread through respiratory drops discharged when a tainted individual hacked or sniffled, and through close contact with discharge-filled skin sores or bedding and other sullied materials.

That was all evident. However, it may not be the entire picture.

More than the vast majority of individuals tainted so far are men who procured the infection through personal contact with different men, as per the Centers for Disease Control and Prevention. Just 13 ladies and two small kids had been determined to have monkeypox as of July 25.

Scientists have tracked down the infection in spit, pee, defecation, and semen. It is hazy whether those liquids can be irresistible and, specifically, whether the infection can be sent during sex by implies other than close skin-to-skin contact. In any case, the example spread up until this point, along with sexual organizations, has left analysts pondering.

It is clear, in any case, that monkeypox doesn't spread effectively and has not yet spilled into the remainder of the populace. The typical individual isn't in danger from locally acquired garments, for instance, or from a transitory connection with a contaminated individual, as a few online entertainment posts have recommended. As indicated by the C.D.C., individuals without side effects can't spread monkeypox. Yet, somewhere around one review has identified the infection in men who encountered no side effects. The example of side effects has likewise separated from that seen in past episodes.

Monkeypox spreads from one individual to another through close contact with somebody who has a monkeypox rash, including through eye to eye, skin-to-skin, mouth-to-mouth, or mouth-to-skin contact, including sexual contact. We are as yet finding out about how long individuals with monkeypox are irresistible, yet for the most part, they are thought of as irresistible until every one of their sores has crusted over, the scabs have tumbled off and another layer of skin has framed under.

Conditions can become debased with the monkeypox infection, for instance when an irresistible individual contacts clothing, bedding, towels, articles, hardware, and surfaces. Another person who contacts these things can then become contaminated. It is additionally conceivable from taking in skin drops or infections from attire, bedding, or towels. This is known as fomite transmission.

Ulcers, sores, or wounds in the mouth can be irresistible, meaning the infection can spread through direct contact with the mouth, respiratory drops, and perhaps through short-range vapor sprayers. Potential instruments of transmission through the air for monkeypox are not yet surely known and studies are in progress to find out more.

The infection can likewise spread from somebody pregnant to the hatchling, after birth through skin-to-skin contact, or from a parent with monkeypox to a baby or kid during close contact.

Although symptomatic contamination has been accounted for, it isn't certain if individuals with no side effects can spread the illness or whether it can spread through other natural liquids. Bits of

DNA from the monkeypox infection have been tracked down in semen, yet it isn't yet known whether the disease can spread through semen, vaginal liquids, amniotic liquids, breastmilk, or blood. Research is in progress to figure out more about whether individuals can spread monkeypox through the trading of these liquids during and after suggestive disease.

Monkeypox can spread to individuals when they come into actual contact with a contaminated creature. The creature has incorporated rodents and primates. The gamble of getting monkeypox from creatures can be decreased by keeping away from unprotected contact with wild creatures, particularly those that are wiped out or dead (counting their meat and blood). In endemic nations where creatures convey monkeypox, any food varieties containing creature meat or parts ought to be cooked completely before eating.

While occurrences of individuals with monkeypox tainting creatures have not been reported, it is a possible gamble. Individuals who have affirmed or thought monkeypox ought to stay away from close contact with creatures, including pets, (for example, felines, canines, hamsters, gerbils, and so on), domesticated animals, and untamed life. Individuals with monkeypox ought to be especially cautious around creatures that are known to be defenceless to the monkeypox infection, including rodents and non-human primates.

AT LAST, MONKEYPOX CAN BE SPREAD THROUGH:

- Direct skin contact with rash injuries

- Sexual/private contact, including kissing

- Residing in a house and imparting a bed to somebody

• Sharing towels or unwashed apparel

• Respiratory emissions through delayed up close and personal corporations (the sort that for the most part happen while living with somebody or focusing on somebody who has monkeypox)

MONKEYPOX IS NOT SPREAD THROUGH:

- Easygoing brief discussions

- Strolling by somebody with monkeypox, as in a supermarket

SYMPTOMS

Monkeypox may produce a variety of signs and symptoms. While some individuals have moderate symptoms, others might develop more significant symptoms and require treatment in a health institution.

Those at increased risk for serious illness or consequences include those who are pregnant. Children and individuals who are immunocompromised.
The most frequent symptoms of monkeypox are fever, headache, muscular discomfort, back pain, poor energy, and enlarged lymph nodes. This is followed or accompanied by the development of a rash which might continue for two to three weeks.

The lash may be found on the face, palms of the hands, soles of the feet, eyes, lips, throat, groin, and genital and/or anal parts of the body. The number of lesions might vary from one to several thousand. Lesions begin flat then fill with fluids until they crust over, dry up and fall off, with a new layer of skin growing behind.

Symptoms normally last two to three weeks and usually go away on their own or with supportive treatment, such as medicine for pain or fever. People stay contagious until all the lesions have crusted over, the scabs come off and a fresh layer of skin has developed below.

Anyone who has symptoms that might be monkeypox or who has been in touch with someone with monkeypox should call or see a health care practitioner and seek their guidance.

In the traditional clinical presentation, monkeypox involves a prodromal phase of fever, malaise, and lymph node enlargement, sometimes with headache and sweating. The lash comes out in two to four days starting as Macules and going on as papules, vesicles, and pustules. These sores gradually scab and fade off.

The lesions arise at the same time predominantly across the face; but, in around 75 percent of patients, lesions will also form over the palms, soles, and mucosa. Genital lesions have been infrequent. Taken collectively, the complete event resolves between two to four weeks.

Complications arise in some people some of which might

include encephalitis, pneumonia, secondary bacterial skin infections, and sight loss owing to eye involvement. Newborn babies and youngsters as well as individuals with compromised immune systems are at a greater risk for complex monkeypox.

However, if you become infected with monkeypox, it normally takes 5 to 21 days for the first signs to develop.

The early signs of monkeypox generally include:

- A high temperature
- A headache
- A muscular soreness
- Backache
- Swollen glands
- Shivering (chills) (chills)
- Exhaustion
- Joint discomfort

A rash normally occurs one to five days after the firmest symptoms. The lash frequently starts on the face, then spreads to other regions of the body. This comprises the mouth, genitals, and anus.

You may also suffer anal discomfort or breeding from your buttock.

The lash is commonly mistaken for chickenpox. It begins as elevated patches, which evolve into little blisters packed with fluid. These blisters gradually produce scabs that subsequently come off.

The adverse effects generally resolve away in half a month. While you suffer side symptoms, you may give monkeypox to others.

PREVENTION

Forestalling the spread of monkeypox

You may help with decreasing your chance of being contaminated with or distributing the monkeypox illness by:

• keeping at home and limiting interaction with people on the off chance that you experience adverse effects, or as recommended by your medical services provider

• keeping away from close physical touch, especially sexual contact, with anybody who is contaminated with or may have been introduced to the monkeypox infection

• keeping up with proper hand cleanliness and respiratory manners, including:

• concealing hacks and sniffles with the twist of your arm or

• wearing a well-fitting cover

• washing and sanitizing high-contact surfaces and things in your house, especially after having visitors

To cut down your general chance of being contaminated with and distributing the monkeypox illness or bodily communicated disorders, we suggest:

• using condoms

• rehearsing safe sex and

• having fewer sexual accomplices, particularly the folks who are unknown, in any case, when they don't have adverse effects

If you believe you could have been contaminated with the monkeypox virus, more deeply study:

• Side consequences of monkeypox contamination

• Getting tried for monkeypox contamination

• Care and treatment presuming you have been found to have monkeypox sickness.

SITUATION SUMMARY

WHAT IS THE TREATMENT FOR MONKEYPOX?

Key realities

• Antibodies employed amid the smallpox annihilation campaign also supplied assurance against monkeypox. More up-to-date antibodies have been produced of which one has been certified for counteraction of monkeypox

• Monkeypox is brought by monkeypox infection, an individual from the Orthopoxvirus type in the family Poxviridae.

• Monkeypox is often a self-restricted illness with the side effects persisting from 2 to around a month. Serious situations may happen. Lately, the case casualty percentage has been at 3-6 percent.

• Monkeypox is conveyed to humans by direct contact with a contaminated person or beast, or through something polluted with the sickness.

• Monkeypox infection is conveyed beginning with one person and then onto the next via intimate contact with injuries, bodily fluid, respiratory beads, and filthy items like sheet material.

• Monkeypox is a viral zoonotic infection that occurs essentially in tropical rainforest regions of focal and west Africa and is at times trafficked to various districts.

• An antiviral specialist created for the therapy of smallpox has likewise been permitted for the treatment of monkeypox.

• The clinical manifestation of monkeypox appears like that of smallpox, a similar orthopoxvirus illness that was announced killed altogether in 1980. Monkeypox is less contagious than smallpox and produces less severe disease.

• Monkeypox commonly appears clinically with fever, rash, and swollen lymph hubs and may trigger a scope of unanticipated complications.

What is the therapy for monkeypox?

The CDC advises the accompanying:

• A smallpox vaccination needs to be controlled in no less than approximately fourteen days of exposure to monkeypox.

• The FDA authorized the Jynneos antibody for vaccination of grown-ups that are at high chance of smallpox or monkeypox (September 2019). (September 2019).

• Cidofovir (Vistide), an antiviral medicine, is advised for people with significant, hazardous adverse effects.

• Vaccinia immune globulin may be employed, however, its effectiveness of usage has not been demonstrated.

For severe symptoms, supporting treatments such as mechanical breathing may infrequently be required. Consultation with an infectious-diseases specialist and the CDC is suggested.

What is the prognosis of monkeypox?

The general prognosis of people with monkeypox is favorable to excellent. Many people experience minimal symptoms. However, individuals with immunological or other weakened health conditions (malnutrition, lung disorders) may experience consequences of secondary bacterial infections, pneumonia, and dehydration.

Older projections of a 10 percent fatality rate were reported, but in the past 10-15 years, this has been lowered to fewer than 2 percent of infected persons, with the deadliest instances arising from the animal-to-human transmission, not person to person.

Is it feasible to prevent monkeypox with a vaccine?

Monkeypox may be avoided by avoiding eating or contacting animals known to get the virus in the wild (primarily African rodents and monkeys) (mainly African rodents and monkeys). The person-to-person transmission has been recorded. Patients who have the illness should physically separate themselves until all of the pox lesions have healed (shed their crusts), and others who are caring for these patients should employ barriers (gloves and face masks) to prevent any direct or droplet contact. Caregivers should acquire a smallpox vaccine.

Because smallpox and monkeypox are so closely related, research has revealed that persons vaccinated against smallpox had around an 85 percent probability of being protected against monkeypox. Consequently, the CDC advises the following:

- Patients with low immune systems and those who are allergic to latex or smallpox immunizations should not have the smallpox vaccine.

- Anyone else who has been exposed to monkeypox in the previous 14 days should obtain the smallpox vaccination, especially children under 1 year of age, pregnant women, and anyone with skin disorders.

There is no commercially available vaccination intended particularly for monkeypox.

What research is being done on monkeypox?

Research is continuing on the monkeypox virus. For example, prairie dogs are being used as animal models to investigate the efficiency of immunizations. Different research is employing animal models to investigate the efficiency of several antiviral medicines to lessen or eliminate symptoms in experimental infections. Because of the close link between smallpox to monkeypox, genetic comparison and genetic change research are anticipated to be accessible in the future, along with more quick detection methods.

What is the incubation time for monkeypox?

The incubation period (time from exposure to first symptoms) is typically seven to 14 days. The early symptoms include fever, headache, muscular aches, swelling lymph nodes, and feeling exhausted. Swollen lymph nodes help differentiate monkeypox from smallpox.

How long is the infectious period for monkeypox?

The sick individual is not infectious throughout the incubation period. However, human instances may be communicable as soon as symptoms begin. The individual is infectious until all scabs from the pox lesions fall off. Consequently, the individual is generally infectious for roughly four to five weeks.

How can health care experts detect monkeypox?

The history (particularly interaction with rats or other animals) and physical exam (presence of pox lesions) provide probable evidence for a diagnosis of monkeypox. Caution is suggested. Infectious disease experts and the Centers for Disease Control and Prevention (CDC) officials should be alerted since this infection may represent two additional issues.

- First, in the U.S. or other countries, it may likely signify an outbreak of monkeypox, and educated health officials may assist to locate the source of the virus and prevent its spread.

- The second concern is improbable but potentially more deadly; the early symptoms may signify biological warfare or terrorist strike using smallpox that is wrongly diagnosed as monkeypox.

Consequently, precise identification of this viral illness, outside of Africa, and particularly in industrialized nations where monkeypox is not prevalent, is advocated. Most laboratories do not have the reagents to undertake this testing, thus state labs or the CDC will need to analyze the samples to make a clear diagnosis. These tests are based on identifying antigenic structures (typically from skin or pox samples or rarely serum) specific to either the monkeypox virus or immunoglobulin that interacts with the virus. PCR (polymerase chain reaction), ELISA procedures (enzyme-linked immunosorbent assay), or Western blotting tests (immunoblotting) are the principal tests employed.

What are the risk factors for monkeypox?

Monkeypox is a very rare illness. Risk factors include animal bites and scratches from infected animals (primarily African rodents or monkeys) or from other rodents (such prairie dogs) that have had contact with African animals infected with the virus. People should avoid consuming any meat from such animals is suggested.

Recent investigations have demonstrated that monkeypox can infect various species of animals, even if the species had never been related to the virus in their usual habitat. Reduce or prevent person-to-person transmission, albeit uncommon, by avoiding direct physical contact with the patient and having the patient's carers use gloves and face masks. Avoid physical contact and clothes with possibly contaminated folks. In Spain, one epidemic (approximately 30 cases) was attributed to a Madrid sauna that is popular with homosexual men. However, monkeypox is not considered a sexually transmitted illness; it may occur more commonly in sexually active populations because of skin-to-skin contact during sex.

www.ingramcontent.com/pod-product-compliance
Lightning Source LLC
LaVergne TN
LVHW052056160826
845678LV00015B/3255

* 9 7 9 8 8 4 4 0 2 6 9 1 1 *